Revitalize Your Body and Mind

A 30-Day Menopause Diet Plan for Weight Loss

Janice R. Dunn

Contents

Copyright

"Revitalize Your Body and Mind: A 30-Day Menopause Diet Plan for Weight Loss"

ISBN: 9798387106316

Imprint: Independently published

Printed in the United States of America

About the author

Janice R. Dunn is a certified nutritionist with over 20 years of experience in the health and wellness industry. She holds

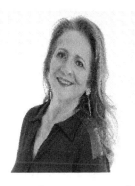

a Master's degree in Nutrition and Dietetics from the University of California, Los Angeles, and is a member of the American Dietetic Association.

Janice's passion for helping women navigate the challenges of menopause led her to create the "Revitalize Your Body and Mind: A 30-Day Menopause Diet for Weight Loss" program. She has helped countless women improve their overall health and well-being by providing practical, evidence-based advice and guidance.

In addition to her work as a nutritionist, Janice is also an avid runner and yogi, and believes that physical activity is essential for maintaining optimal health and wellness. She resides in Los Angeles, California, with her husband and two children.

Preface

Welcome to "Revitalize Your Body and Mind: A 30-Day Menopause Diet for Weight Loss," a comprehensive guide to managing the symptoms of menopause and achieving optimal health and wellness. As a certified nutritionist with over 20 years of experience in the health and wellness industry, I understand the challenges that women face during this transitional period in their lives.

This book is a result of my passion for helping women navigate through the challenges of menopause and make positive changes to their diets and lifestyles. By providing evidence-based advice and practical guidance, I hope to empower women to take control of their health and make informed decisions about their diet and lifestyle choices.

Throughout this book, you will find a 30-day meal plan specifically designed to help women going through menopause lose weight and manage their symptoms. Additionally, you will learn about the importance of exercise, mindfulness, and self-care during menopause, and how to incorporate these practices into your daily routine.

I want to thank you for taking the time to invest in your health and well-being. I hope that this book will serve as a valuable resource to help you achieve your health and wellness goals. Remember, small changes can lead to big results, and with dedication and perseverance, you can revitalize your body and mind during this important stage of your life.

A 30-Day Menopause Diet Plan for Weight Loss

Best, Janice R. Dunn, MS, RD, CDN.

Chapter 1. Introduction

Menopause is a natural transition in a woman's life that marks the end of her reproductive years. It's a process that occurs gradually, typically starting in a woman's 40s or 50s, but can happen earlier or later than that.

During menopause, a woman's body undergoes significant hormonal changes. One of the most well-known symptoms of menopause is hot flashes, which affect around 75% of women. Hot flashes can be extremely uncomfortable and can disrupt sleep, making it more difficult to manage other menopause symptoms.

In addition to hot flashes, many women experience other symptoms during menopause, such as mood swings, vaginal dryness, and decreased sex drive. These symptoms can be frustrating and difficult to manage, and they can have a significant impact on a woman's quality of life.

But menopause can also have more serious effects on a woman's health. For example, women going through menopause are at an increased risk for heart disease, which is the leading cause of death for women in the United States. In fact, women's risk of heart disease increases significantly after menopause, with some studies suggesting that women's risk of heart disease doubles within 10 years of menopause.

Menopause can also lead to a decrease in bone density, which puts women at risk for osteoporosis and fractures. In fact, women can lose up to 20% of their bone mass in the 5-7 years following menopause, putting them at increased risk for fractures.

Another common effect of menopause is weight gain. As hormone levels change, women may experience an increase in belly fat, which can be difficult to lose. In fact, one study found that women gain an average of 1.5 pounds per year during menopause.

Understanding the effects of menopause on the body is crucial in developing an effective menopause diet for weight loss. By nourishing your body with the right foods and supplements, you can mitigate the negative effects of menopause and feel your best during this important stage of life.

The Benefits of a Menopause Diet for Weight Loss

Many women going through menopause struggle with weight gain and find it difficult to lose the extra pounds. But did you know that following a menopause diet for weight loss can have a range of benefits beyond just shedding unwanted pounds?

One of the biggest benefits of a menopause diet for weight loss is that it can help reduce the risk of chronic diseases. As women go through menopause, their risk of heart disease, osteoporosis, and other chronic conditions increases. But by following a healthy diet that is rich in fruits, vegetables, whole grains, and lean proteins, women can lower their risk of these diseases and improve their overall health.

In addition to reducing the risk of chronic diseases, a menopause diet for weight loss can also help alleviate menopause symptoms. For example, eating foods that are high in phytoestrogens, such as soybeans and flaxseeds, can help alleviate hot flashes and other symptoms by mimicking the effects of estrogen in the body. Similarly, consuming foods that are high in calcium and vitamin D can help prevent bone loss and reduce the risk of osteoporosis.

But the benefits of a menopause diet for weight loss don't stop there. Eating a healthy diet can also improve mood and cognitive function, which can be especially important during menopause when women may experience mood swings and brain fog. And, of course, losing weight can also improve self-confidence and body image, which can have a positive impact on the overall quality of life.

Following a menopause diet for weight loss can have numerous benefits for women going through this important life transition. By nourishing the body with healthy and nutritious foods, women can improve their overall health, reduce the risk of chronic diseases, alleviate menopause symptoms, and feel their best during this time of change.

Overview of the 30-Day Menopause Diet Plan

The 30-Day Menopause Diet Plan is designed to help women going through menopause lose weight, manage symptoms, and improve overall health and well-being. The plan is broken down into four weeks, each with a specific focus and meal plan.

Week 1: Cleanse and Reset During the first week, the focus is on cleansing the body and resetting the digestive system. This is achieved through a combination of nutrient-dense foods and a reduction in processed foods and sugar. The meal plan includes plenty of fruits and vegetables, lean proteins, and healthy fats. This week sets the foundation for the rest of the plan.

Week 2: Boost Metabolism The second week is all about boosting metabolism and increasing energy levels. This is achieved through a higher protein intake, which helps to increase metabolism and support muscle mass. The meal plan includes plenty of lean proteins, such as chicken, fish, and tofu, as well as healthy fats and whole grains.

Week 3: Reduce Inflammation Inflammation can contribute to a range of health issues, including chronic diseases and menopause symptoms. During the third week, the focus is on reducing inflammation through a diet rich in anti-inflammatory foods, such as leafy greens, berries, and fatty fish. The meal plan includes plenty of colorful fruits and vegetables, healthy fats, and lean proteins.

Week 4: Maintain and Sustain The final week of the plan is all about maintaining weight loss and sustaining healthy habits for the long term. This week focuses on a well-balanced diet that includes a variety of foods, including lean proteins, whole grains, fruits and vegetables, and healthy fats. The meal plan is designed to be sustainable and enjoyable so that women can continue to follow healthy eating habits beyond the 30 days.

Throughout the 30-Day Menopause Diet Plan, you will also find tips for success, such as how to meal prep and plan ahead, as well as strategies for overcoming barriers to success. By following the plan and making healthy choices, you can achieve your weight loss and health goals during menopause and beyond.

Chapter 2. Managing Menopause Symptoms with Diet

Menopause is a natural transition in a woman's life that marks the end of her reproductive years. During menopause, a woman's body undergoes significant hormonal changes that can lead to a variety of symptoms. Some of the most common menopause symptoms include:

Hot flashes: Hot flashes are characterized by a sudden feeling of heat that spreads across the body, often accompanied by sweating and chills. They can last from a few seconds to several minutes, and can be extremely uncomfortable.

Night sweats: Night sweats are similar to hot flashes, but they occur during sleep and can disrupt sleep, leading to fatigue and other symptoms.

Mood swings: Many women experience mood swings during menopause, ranging from irritability and anxiety to depression and feelings of sadness.

Vaginal dryness: The hormonal changes during menopause can lead to a decrease in vaginal lubrication, which can cause discomfort and pain during sex.

Decreased sex drive: The decrease in estrogen during menopause can also lead to a decrease in sex drive, which can impact a woman's quality of life.

Difficulty sleeping: Sleep disturbances are common during menopause, with many women experiencing difficulty falling asleep or staying asleep.

Weight gain: Hormonal changes during menopause can lead to weight gain, particularly in the abdominal area.

It's important to note that not all women experience the same symptoms during menopause, and the severity of symptoms can vary widely. However, understanding common menopause symptoms can help women prepare for this important life transition and find ways to manage their symptoms. In the following chapters, we'll explore how a menopause diet for weight loss can help alleviate these symptoms and improve overall health and well-being.

Foods to Eat and Avoid for Symptom Management

Eating a healthy and balanced diet is important for managing menopause symptoms and improving overall health and well-being. Here are some foods to eat and avoid for symptom management during menopause:

Foods to Eat:

1. Fruits and Vegetables: Eating a variety of colorful fruits and vegetables can provide essential vitamins, minerals, and fiber, which can help manage menopause symptoms. Aim for at least five servings per day.
2. Whole Grains: Whole grains, such as brown rice, quinoa, and oats, can provide energy and fiber,

which can help regulate digestion and reduce hot flashes.

3. Lean Proteins: Eating lean proteins, such as chicken, fish, tofu, and beans, can help maintain muscle mass and boost metabolism. It can also provide essential nutrients for overall health.

4. Calcium-rich Foods: Women going through menopause are at an increased risk for osteoporosis, so it's important to consume plenty of calcium-rich foods, such as dairy products, leafy greens, and fortified plant-based milks.

5. Phytoestrogen-rich Foods: Phytoestrogens are compounds found in certain foods, such as soybeans, flaxseeds, and chickpeas, that mimic the effects of estrogen in the body. Consuming these foods can help alleviate hot flashes and other symptoms.

Foods to Avoid:

1. Processed Foods: Processed foods can be high in sugar, sodium, and unhealthy fats, which can contribute to weight gain and other health issues. It's important to limit processed foods and focus on whole, nutrient-dense foods instead.

2. Caffeine and Alcohol: Both caffeine and alcohol can disrupt sleep and contribute to hot flashes and other symptoms. It's important to limit or avoid these beverages to manage menopause symptoms.

3. Spicy Foods: Spicy foods can trigger hot flashes and other symptoms, so it's important to avoid them or limit their consumption.

4. High-fat Foods: High-fat foods, particularly those high in saturated and trans fats, can contribute to weight gain and other health issues. It's important to limit these foods and focus on healthier fats, such as those found in nuts, seeds, and avocados.

By incorporating these foods into a menopause diet for weight loss, you can manage their symptoms and improve overall health and well-being.

Recipes and Meal Ideas for Symptom Relief

One of the most important aspects of a menopause diet for weight loss is ensuring that the foods we eat are nutrient-dense and provide us with the necessary vitamins and minerals to manage menopause symptoms. By incorporating a variety of whole, healthy foods into our diet, we can reduce inflammation, regulate digestion, and improve overall health and well-being.

Here are some recipes and meal ideas for symptom relief during menopause:

1. Breakfast Smoothie Bowl: Blend together frozen berries, spinach, Greek yogurt, and a splash of almond milk for a nutritious and delicious smoothie bowl. Top with sliced banana, granola, and chia seeds for added texture and flavor.

2. Roasted Vegetable Salad: Roast a variety of vegetables, such as sweet potato, zucchini, bell

peppers, and Brussels sprouts, and serve over a bed of mixed greens. Drizzle with balsamic vinaigrette and top with grilled chicken or tofu for a filling and nutrient-packed meal.

3. Quinoa and Black Bean Bowl: Cook quinoa and black beans according to package instructions and serve with sautéed onions and bell peppers, avocado, and a squeeze of lime. This meal is high in protein and fiber, which can help manage menopause symptoms.

4. Grilled Chicken with Cauliflower Rice: Grill a chicken breast and serve with cauliflower rice, which can be made by pulsing cauliflower in a food processor. Add chopped vegetables, such as carrots and peas, for added nutrition and flavor.

5. Dark Chocolate-Covered Strawberries: For a healthy and satisfying dessert, dip strawberries in melted dark chocolate and sprinkle with chopped nuts or shredded coconut. Dark chocolate is high in antioxidants, which can help reduce inflammation and manage menopause symptoms.

Chapter 3. Mindful Eating

Mindful eating is an important aspect of a menopausal diet for weight loss. It involves being fully present and engaged in the eating experience, paying attention to the tastes, smells, and textures of the food we eat. By practicing mindful eating, we can become more attuned to our body's hunger and fullness signals, and make more conscious and healthy food choices.

One of the key benefits of mindful eating is that it can help prevent overeating and emotional eating, which can be common during menopause. By taking the time to truly savor our food and listen to our body's signals, we can avoid mindless snacking and make more mindful choices that support our health and well-being.

In addition to helping manage weight, mindful eating can also reduce stress and promote relaxation. By focusing on the present moment and being fully engaged in the eating experience, we can reduce feelings of anxiety and tension, which can be beneficial during menopause when mood swings and stress can be common.

Techniques for Practicing Mindful Eating

Here's an overview of some techniques for practicing mindful eating:

1. Slow Down: One of the simplest ways to practice mindful eating is to slow down while eating. Take small bites, chew your food thoroughly, and savor

each bite. This will help you become more aware of the flavors and textures of your food, and can help you feel more satisfied and full.

2. Eliminate Distractions: When eating, eliminate distractions such as TV, social media, and work. Instead, focus on the food in front of you and the experience of eating. This can help you be more present in the moment and enjoy your food more fully.

3. Pay Attention to Hunger and Fullness: Pay attention to your body's hunger and fullness signals while eating. Stop eating when you feel full, even if there is food left on your plate. This can help prevent overeating and promote mindful choices.

4. Use All Your Senses: Engage all your senses while eating. Notice the colors, smells, textures, and tastes of your food. This can help you appreciate the food more and make more mindful choices.

5. Practice Gratitude: Before eating, take a moment to express gratitude for the food on your plate and the experience of eating. This can help you feel more positive and mindful during the meal.

Incorporating these techniques into your menopause diet for weight loss can help you become more mindful and conscious of your eating habits. By practicing mindful eating, you can manage menopause symptoms, reduce stress, and promote overall health and well-being. With the help of these techniques, you can savor your meals more fully, avoid overeating, and make healthier food choices that support your health goals.

Mindful Eating and Menopause

During menopause, hormonal changes can lead to a variety of physical and emotional symptoms, including weight gain, hot flashes, mood swings, and fatigue. These symptoms can be exacerbated by unhealthy eating habits and emotional eating, which can lead to further weight gain and a decrease in overall health and well-being.

Practicing mindful eating can be particularly beneficial during menopause, as it can help manage symptoms and promote overall health and well-being. By becoming more aware of our eating habits and paying closer attention to our body's signals, we can make more conscious and healthy choices that support our health goals.

Mindful eating can help manage menopause symptoms in a variety of ways. By eating slowly and savoring each bite, we can reduce stress and promote relaxation, which can help manage mood swings and other emotional symptoms. Paying attention to hunger and fullness signals can also help prevent overeating and weight gain, which can be common during menopause.

In addition to managing symptoms, practicing mindful eating can promote overall health and well-being during menopause. By focusing on nutrient-dense whole foods and eliminating distractions during meals, we can improve digestion, increase energy levels, and reduce inflammation in the body.

Chapter 4. Week 1: Cleanse and Reset

Week 1 of the 30-day Menopause Diet for Weight Loss is all about cleansing and resetting your body to kickstart your weight loss journey. During this week, we'll focus on eliminating processed foods, sugar, and alcohol from your diet and replacing them with nutrient-dense whole foods that support your health and well-being.

The cleanse and reset week is designed to help jumpstart your metabolism, reduce inflammation in your body, and improve your digestion. By following the daily meal plan and practicing mindful eating, you can become more aware of your eating habits and make healthier choices that support your health goals.

In addition to the daily meal plan, it's important to stay hydrated by drinking plenty of water throughout the day. You can also incorporate gentle exercise and stress-reducing activities such as yoga, meditation, or deep breathing to support your cleanse and reset process.

Remember, Week 1 is just the beginning of your 30-day journey. By focusing on nutrient-dense whole foods and practicing mindful eating, you can improve your health and well-being and kickstart your weight loss journey.

Daily Meal Plan
Here's a day-by-day breakdown of the Week 1 meal plan:

Day 1

Breakfast:

- Greek yogurt with sliced strawberries, walnuts, and honey
- Green smoothie with spinach, frozen peaches, almond milk, and protein powder

Snack:

- Carrot sticks with hummus
- Handful of almonds

Lunch:

- Grilled chicken salad with mixed greens, cherry tomatoes, cucumber, and balsamic vinaigrette
- Quinoa and black bean bowl with sautéed onions and peppers, avocado, and a squeeze of lime

Snack:

- Greek yogurt with mixed berries and granola
- Hard-boiled egg with salt and pepper

Dinner:

- Grilled shrimp with roasted asparagus and sweet potato wedges
- Zucchini noodles with tomato sauce and Parmesan cheese

Snack:

- Dark chocolate-covered strawberries

- Sliced pear with cinnamon and ricotta cheese

Day 2

Breakfast:

- Chia seed pudding with almond milk, sliced banana, and cinnamon
- Green smoothie with kale, frozen mango, almond milk, and protein powder

Snack:

- Apple slices with almond butter
- Handful of cashews

Lunch:

- Turkey burger with mixed greens, sliced tomato, and avocado on a whole-grain bun
- Quinoa and black bean bowl with sautéed onions and peppers, avocado, and a squeeze of lime

Snack:

- Greek yogurt with mixed berries and granola
- Baby carrots with hummus

Dinner:

- Broiled salmon with roasted Brussels sprouts and sweet potato wedges
- Cauliflower rice with stir-fried mixed vegetables

Snack:

- Dark chocolate-covered almonds
- Sliced pear with cinnamon and ricotta cheese

Day 3

Breakfast:

- Oatmeal with sliced banana, almond milk, and cinnamon
- Green smoothie with spinach, frozen mixed berries, almond milk, and protein powder

Snack:

- Handful of almonds
- Sliced apple with peanut butter

Lunch:

- Chicken and veggie stir-fry with brown rice
- Grilled vegetable salad with mixed greens and balsamic vinaigrette

Snack:

- Greek yogurt with mixed berries and granola
- Carrot sticks with hummus

Dinner:

- Grilled chicken breast with roasted asparagus and sweet potato wedges

- Quinoa and black bean bowl with sautéed onions and peppers, avocado, and a squeeze of lime

Snack:

- Dark chocolate-covered strawberries
- Sliced pear with cinnamon and ricotta cheese

Day 4

Breakfast:

- Scrambled eggs with sautéed spinach, sliced avocado, and whole-grain toast
- Green smoothie with kale, frozen pineapple, almond milk, and protein powder

Snack:

- Handful of cashews
- Sliced apple with almond butter

Lunch:

- Grilled salmon with mixed greens, cherry tomatoes, cucumber, and balsamic vinaigrette
- Quinoa and black bean bowl with sautéed onions and peppers, avocado, and a squeeze of lime

Snack:

- Greek yogurt with mixed berries and granola
- Baby carrots with hummus

Dinner:

- Grilled chicken skewers with mixed vegetables and quinoa
- Cauliflower rice with stir-fried mixed vegetables

Snack:

- Dark chocolate-covered almonds
- Sliced pear with cinnamon and ricotta cheese

Day 5

Breakfast:

- Greek yogurt with sliced peaches, cashews, and honey
- Green smoothie with spinach, frozen strawberries, almond milk, and protein powder

Snack:

- Carrot sticks with hummus
- Handful of almonds

Lunch:

- Grilled chicken salad with mixed greens, cherry tomatoes, cucumber, and balsamic vinaigrette
- Quinoa and black bean bowl with sautéed onions and peppers, avocado, and a squeeze of lime

Snack:

- Greek yogurt with mixed berries and granola
- Hard-boiled egg with salt and pepper

Dinner:

- Baked salmon with roasted broccoli and sweet potato wedges
- Zucchini noodles with tomato sauce and Parmesan cheese

Snack:

- Dark chocolate-covered strawberries
- Sliced pear with cinnamon and ricotta cheese

Day 6

Breakfast:

- Omelette with spinach, sliced tomato, and feta cheese
- Green smoothie with kale, frozen blueberries, almond milk, and protein powder

Snack:

- Apple slices with almond butter
- Handful of cashews

Lunch:

- Turkey burger with mixed greens, sliced tomato, and avocado on a whole-grain bun
- Quinoa and black bean bowl with sautéed onions and peppers, avocado, and a squeeze of lime

Snack:

- Greek yogurt with mixed berries and granola
- Baby carrots with hummus

Dinner:

- Grilled chicken breast with roasted Brussels sprouts and sweet potato wedges
- Cauliflower rice with stir-fried mixed vegetables

Snack:

- Dark chocolate-covered almonds
- Sliced pear with cinnamon and ricotta cheese

Day 7

Breakfast:

- Chia seed pudding with almond milk, sliced banana, and cinnamon
- Green smoothie with spinach, frozen mixed berries, almond milk, and protein powder

Snack:

- Handful of almonds
- Sliced apple with peanut butter

Lunch:

- Chicken and veggie stir-fry with brown rice

- Grilled vegetable salad with mixed greens and balsamic vinaigrette

Snack:

- Greek yogurt with mixed berries and granola
- Carrot sticks with hummus

Dinner:

- Grilled salmon with mixed greens, cherry tomatoes, cucumber, and balsamic vinaigrette
- Quinoa and black bean bowl with sautéed onions and peppers, avocado, and a squeeze of lime

Snack:

- Dark chocolate-covered strawberries
- Sliced pear with cinnamon and ricotta cheese

Remember, you can always adjust these meal plans to fit your individual needs and preferences. The key is to focus on nutrient-dense whole foods and eliminate processed foods and sugar during Week 1. Drinking plenty of water and practicing mindful eating can also help support the cleanse and reset process.

Recipes and Meal Ideas

Here are some recipes and meal ideas for Week 1: Cleanse and Reset of the menopause diet for weight loss:

Grilled Shrimp with Roasted Asparagus and Sweet Potato Wedges

Ingredients

- 4 oz. shrimp, peeled and deveined
- 1/2 bunch asparagus, trimmed
- 1 medium sweet potato, cut into wedges
- 1 tbsp olive oil
- Salt and pepper to taste

Directions:

1. Preheat the oven to 400°F.
2. Toss the sweet potato wedges with olive oil, salt, and pepper.
3. Place the sweet potato wedges in a single layer on a baking sheet and roast for 20-25 minutes or until tender.
4. Preheat a grill or grill pan over medium-high heat.
5. Season the shrimp with salt and pepper and grill for 2-3 minutes per side or until cooked through.
6. Grill the asparagus for 3-4 minutes or until tender.
7. Serve the shrimp with the roasted sweet potato wedges and grilled asparagus.

Chicken and Veggie Stir-Fry with Brown Rice

Ingredients

- 4 oz. boneless, skinless chicken breast, sliced
- 1 cup mixed vegetables (e.g. bell pepper, onion, broccoli)
- 1 clove garlic, minced
- 1 tbsp soy sauce
- 1 tsp cornstarch

- 1/2 cup cooked brown rice

Directions:

1. Heat a wok or large skillet over medium-high heat.
2. Add the chicken and stir-fry for 2-3 minutes or until browned.
3. Add the mixed vegetables and garlic and stir-fry for an additional 2-3 minutes or until tender.
4. In a small bowl, whisk together the soy sauce and cornstarch.
5. Pour the soy sauce mixture over the chicken and vegetables and stir to combine.
6. Cook for an additional 1-2 minutes or until the sauce thickens.
7. Serve over cooked brown rice.

Broiled Salmon with Roasted Asparagus and Sweet Potato Wedges

Ingredients

- 4 oz. salmon fillet
- 1/2 bunch asparagus, trimmed
- 1 medium sweet potato, cut into wedges
- 1 tbsp olive oil
- Salt and pepper to taste

Directions:

1. Preheat the oven to 400°F.

2. Toss the sweet potato wedges with olive oil, salt, and pepper.
3. Place the sweet potato wedges in a single layer on a baking sheet and roast for 20-25 minutes or until tender.
4. Preheat the broiler to high.
5. Season the salmon with salt and pepper and place on a baking sheet.
6. Broil the salmon for 5-7 minutes or until cooked through.
7. Grill the asparagus for 3-4 minutes or until tender.
8. Serve the salmon with the roasted sweet potato wedges and grilled asparagus.

Baked Chicken with Roasted Broccoli and Sweet Potato Wedges

Ingredients:

- 4 oz. chicken breast
- 1 cup broccoli florets
- 1 medium sweet potato, cut into wedges
- 1 tbsp olive oil
- Salt and pepper to taste

Directions:

1. Preheat the oven to 400°F.
2. Toss the sweet potato wedges with olive oil, salt, and pepper.

3. Place the sweet potato wedges in a single layer on a baking sheet and roast for 20-25 minutes or until tender.
4. Place the chicken breast on the same baking sheet and season with salt and pepper.
5. Bake for 20-25 minutes or until the chicken is cooked through and the juices run clear.
6. In the last 10 minutes of cooking, add the broccoli florets to the baking sheet and toss with olive oil, salt, and pepper.
7. Serve the baked chicken with the roasted sweet potato wedges and broccoli.

Greek Yogurt Parfait with Berries and Almonds

Ingredients

- 1/2 cup plain Greek yogurt
- 1/2 cup mixed berries (e.g., strawberries, blueberries, raspberries)
- 1/4 cup sliced almonds
- 1 tsp honey (optional)

Directions:

1. Layer the Greek yogurt, mixed berries, and sliced almonds in a parfait glass or bowl.
2. Drizzle with honey if desired.

4 oz. sirloin steak

Ingredients

- 1/2 bunch asparagus, trimmed
- 1 cup cauliflower rice
- 1 tbsp olive oil
- Salt and pepper to taste

Directions:

1. Preheat the oven to 400°F.
2. Place the cauliflower rice on a baking sheet and toss it with olive oil, salt, and pepper.
3. Roast the cauliflower rice for 15-20 minutes or until tender.
4. Preheat a grill or grill pan over medium-high heat.
5. Season the steak with salt and pepper and grill for 4-5 minutes per side or until cooked to your desired doneness.
6. Grill the asparagus for 3-4 minutes or until tender.
7. Serve the grilled steak with the roasted cauliflower rice and asparagus.

Grilled Salmon with Roasted Vegetables

Ingredients

- 4 oz. salmon fillet
- 1/2 cup chopped broccoli
- 1/2 cup chopped cauliflower
- 1/2 cup chopped carrots

- 1 tbsp olive oil
- Salt and pepper to taste

Directions:

1. Preheat the oven to 400°F.
2. Toss the vegetables with olive oil, salt, and pepper.
3. Place the vegetables in a single layer on a baking sheet and roast for 20-25 minutes or until tender.
4. Preheat a grill or grill pan over medium-high heat.
5. Season the salmon with salt and pepper and grill for 3-4 minutes per side or until cooked through.
6. Serve the salmon with the roasted vegetables.

Quinoa and Black Bean Bowl

Ingredients

- 1/2 cup cooked quinoa
- 1/2 cup black beans, drained and rinsed
- 1/2 cup diced tomatoes
- 1/4 cup diced red onion
- 1/4 cup diced bell pepper
- 1/4 cup diced avocado
- Juice of 1 lime
- Salt and pepper to taste

Directions:

1. Combine the quinoa, black beans, tomatoes, red onion, bell pepper, and avocado in a bowl.

2. Squeeze the lime juice over the bowl and toss to combine.
3. Season with salt and pepper to taste.

Grilled Chicken Salad

Ingredients

- 4 oz. grilled chicken breast
- 2 cups mixed greens
- 1/2 cup cherry tomatoes
- 1/4 cup sliced cucumber
- 1/4 cup sliced red onion
- 2 tbsp balsamic vinaigrette

Directions:

1. Toss the mixed greens, cherry tomatoes, cucumber, and red onion in a bowl.
2. Top with the grilled chicken breast.
3. Drizzle with the balsamic vinaigrette.

Remember, these are just a few examples of the delicious and healthy meals you can enjoy during Week 1. Feel free to mix and match these recipes to create your own meal plan that suits your individual tastes and preferences. And don't forget to drink plenty of water and practice mindful eating throughout the day!

Tips for Success

To help ensure success during Week 1 of the 30-day Menopause Diet for Weight Loss, here are some tips to keep in mind:

1. Plan ahead: Take some time at the beginning of the week to plan your meals and snacks for the upcoming days. This can help you avoid impulsive food choices and ensure that you have healthy options available when hunger strikes.
2. Stock up on healthy foods: Make sure your kitchen is stocked with nutrient-dense whole foods such as vegetables, fruits, lean proteins, and healthy fats. This can help you resist the temptation to reach for unhealthy processed foods when hunger strikes.
3. Practice mindful eating: During Week 1, focus on eating slowly and mindfully. Pay attention to your body's hunger and fullness cues, and take time to savor each bite of your meals.
4. Stay hydrated: Drinking plenty of water throughout the day can help you feel fuller and more satisfied, and can also help support your body's natural detoxification processes.
5. Incorporate gentle exercise: During Week 1, aim to incorporate some gentle exercise into your daily routine. This can help boost your metabolism and support your body's natural detoxification processes.

When you follow these tips and commit to the 30-day Menopause Diet for Weight Loss, you can kickstart your weight loss journey and improve your overall health and well-being. Remember, every small step counts towards your success!

Chapter 5. Week 2: Boost Metabolism

Week 2 of the 30-day Menopause Diet for Weight Loss is all about boosting your metabolism to help burn more calories and support your weight loss goals. During this week, we'll focus on incorporating metabolism-boosting foods into your diet and incorporating more physical activity into your daily routine.

By increasing your metabolism, you can help your body burn more calories even when you're at rest. This can help you achieve your weight loss goals more quickly and efficiently.

In addition to the daily meal plan, it's important to stay active during Week 2. Incorporating more physical activity into your daily routine can help increase your metabolism and support your weight loss goals. Try going for a brisk walk, taking a yoga class, or trying a new workout routine to get your body moving.

Remember, Week 2 is all about boosting your metabolism to support your weight loss goals. By following the daily meal plan and staying active, you can help support your body's natural ability to burn calories and achieve your desired weight.

Daily Meal Plan

Day 8:

Breakfast

- Greek yogurt with mixed berries and sliced almonds

Snack

- Apple slices with almond butter

Lunch

- Turkey and avocado wrap with mixed greens

Snack

- Carrots and hummus

Dinner

- Grilled chicken with roasted Brussels sprouts and quinoa

Day 9:

Breakfast

- Spinach and mushroom omelette with whole wheat toast

Snack

- Plain Greek yogurt with sliced bananas and honey

Lunch

- Tuna salad with mixed greens and whole grain crackers

Snack

- Celery sticks with peanut butter

Dinner

- Grilled salmon with roasted asparagus and sweet potato wedges

Day 10:

Breakfast

- Blueberry smoothie bowl with chia seeds and granola

Snack

- Cottage cheese with diced pineapple

Lunch

- Chicken and vegetable stir-fry with brown rice

Snack

- Edamame pods

Dinner

- Beef and vegetable kebabs with quinoa salad

Day 11:

Breakfast

- Oatmeal with mixed berries and sliced almonds

Snack

- Hard-boiled egg with sliced cucumbers

Lunch

- Grilled shrimp and vegetable skewers with mixed greens

Snack

- Sliced pear with goat cheese

Dinner

- Baked chicken with roasted broccoli and cauliflower rice

Day 12:

Breakfast

- Greek yogurt with mixed berries, chia seeds, and honey

Snack

- Sliced apple with peanut butter

Lunch

- Turkey burger with sweet potato fries and mixed greens

Snack

- Carrots and hummus

Dinner

- Grilled chicken with roasted cauliflower and brown rice

Day 13:

Breakfast

- Spinach and feta omelette with whole wheat toast

Snack

- Cottage cheese with sliced peaches

Lunch

- Shrimp and vegetable stir-fry with brown rice

Snack

- Edamame pods

Dinner

- Baked salmon with roasted Brussels sprouts and quinoa

Day 14:

Breakfast

- Blueberry smoothie with almond milk and protein powder

Snack

- Hard-boiled egg with sliced cucumbers

Lunch

- Grilled chicken Caesar salad with whole grain croutons

Snack

- Sliced pear with almond butter

Dinner

- Grilled steak with roasted asparagus and sweet potato wedges

Mix and match these meal ideas to suit your individual preferences and tastes. And don't forget to stay hydrated by drinking plenty of water throughout the day!

Recipes and Meal Ideas

Here are some of the recipe ideas with ingredient lists based on the foods listed in the day-by-day breakdown of the Week 2 meal plan:

Grilled Chicken with Roasted Brussels Sprouts and Quinoa

Ingredients:

- 4 boneless, skinless chicken breasts
- 1/4 cup olive oil
- 1/4 cup lemon juice
- 2 garlic cloves, minced
- 1 teaspoon dried oregano
- Salt and pepper to taste
- 1 pound Brussels sprouts, trimmed and halved
- 2 tablespoons olive oil
- Salt and pepper to taste
- 1 cup quinoa
- 2 cups water or low-sodium chicken broth

Directions:

1. In a large bowl, whisk together the olive oil, lemon juice, garlic, oregano, salt, and pepper.
2. Add the chicken breasts to the bowl and toss to coat. Let marinate for at least 30 minutes, or up to 24 hours in the refrigerator.
3. Preheat the grill to medium heat. Remove the chicken from the marinade and discard any excess marinade.

4. Grill the chicken for 6-8 minutes per side, until cooked through.
5. Meanwhile, preheat the oven to 400°F. Toss the Brussels sprouts with olive oil, salt, and pepper, and spread them in a single layer on a baking sheet. Roast for 25-30 minutes, until tender and lightly browned.
6. Cook the quinoa according to package instructions.
7. Serve the grilled chicken with the roasted Brussels sprouts and cooked quinoa.

Shrimp and Vegetable Stir-Fry with Brown Rice

Ingredients:

-   1 pound raw shrimp, peeled and deveined
-   2 tablespoons olive oil
-   3 cloves garlic, minced
-   1 tablespoon grated ginger
-   2 tablespoons low-sodium soy sauce
-   1 red bell pepper, thinly sliced
-   2 carrots, thinly sliced
-   1 cup snow peas
-   2 cups cooked brown rice

Directions:

1. In a large skillet or wok, heat the olive oil over medium-high heat. Add the garlic and ginger and sauté for 1-2 minutes, until fragrant.

2. Add the shrimp to the pan and cook for 3-5 minutes, until pink and cooked through.
3. Add the sliced bell pepper, carrots, and snow peas to the pan and cook for an additional 5-7 minutes, until the vegetables are tender-crisp.
4. Stir in the soy sauce and cook for 1-2 minutes to heat through.
5. Serve the shrimp and vegetable stir-fry over the cooked brown rice.

Grilled Steak with Roasted Sweet Potato Wedges and Mixed Greens

Ingredients:

- 4 boneless ribeye or sirloin steaks
- 1/4 cup olive oil
- 1/4 cup balsamic vinegar
- 2 garlic cloves, minced
- 1 tablespoon chopped fresh rosemary
- Salt and pepper to taste
- 2 large sweet potatoes, cut into wedges
- 2 tablespoons olive oil
- 1 teaspoon paprika
- Salt and pepper to taste
- 4 cups mixed greens
- Balsamic vinaigrette for dressing

Directions:

1. In a large bowl, whisk together the olive oil, balsamic vinegar, garlic, rosemary, salt, and pepper.
2. Add the steaks to the bowl and toss to coat. Let marinate for at least 30 minutes, or up to 24 hours in the refrigerator.
3. Preheat the grill to medium-high heat. Remove the steaks from the marinade and discard any excess marinade.
4. Grill the steaks for 4-5 minutes per side for medium-rare, or longer to your desired level of doneness.
5. Meanwhile, preheat the oven to 400°F. Toss the sweet potato wedges with olive oil, paprika, salt, and pepper, and spread them in a single layer on a baking sheet. Roast for 25-30 minutes, until tender and lightly browned.
6. Toss the mixed greens with balsamic vinaigrette and divide among four plates.
7. Serve the grilled steak with the roasted sweet potato wedges and mixed greens.

Chicken with Roasted Brussels Sprouts and Quinoa

Ingredients:

1. 4 boneless, skinless chicken breasts
2. 1/4 cup olive oil
3. 1/4 cup lemon juice
4. 2 garlic cloves, minced
5. 1 teaspoon dried oregano Salt and pepper to taste
6. 1 pound Brussels sprouts, trimmed and halved

7. 2 tablespoons olive oil Salt and pepper to taste
8. 1 cup quinoa
9. 2 cups water or low-sodium chicken broth

Directions:

1. In a large bowl, whisk together the olive oil, lemon juice, garlic, oregano, salt, and pepper.
2. Add the chicken breasts to the bowl and toss to coat. Let marinate for at least 30 minutes, or up to 24 hours in the refrigerator.
3. Preheat the grill to medium heat. Remove the chicken from the marinade and discard any excess marinade.
4. Grill the chicken for 6-8 minutes per side, until cooked through.
5. Meanwhile, preheat the oven to 400°F. Toss the Brussels sprouts with olive oil, salt, and pepper, and spread them in a single layer on a baking sheet. Roast for 25-30 minutes, until tender and lightly browned.
6. Cook the quinoa according to package instructions.
7. Serve the grilled chicken with the roasted Brussels sprouts and cooked quinoa.

Grilled Turkey Burgers with Sweet Potato Fries and Salad

Ingredients:

- 1 pound ground turkey
- 1/4 cup diced red onion

- 1/4 cup chopped fresh parsley
- 2 cloves garlic, minced
- 1 teaspoon ground cumin
- Salt and pepper to taste
- 4 whole wheat hamburger buns
- 1 large sweet potato, cut into fries
- 2 tablespoons olive oil
- Salt and pepper to taste
- 4 cups mixed greens
- Dressing of choice

Directions:

1. In a large bowl, combine the ground turkey, red onion, parsley, garlic, cumin, salt, and pepper. Mix well and form into four patties.
2. Preheat the grill to medium-high heat. Grill the turkey burgers for 4-5 minutes per side, until cooked through.
3. Meanwhile, preheat the oven to 425°F. Toss the sweet potato fries with olive oil, salt, and pepper, and spread them in a single layer on a baking sheet. Roast for 20-25 minutes, until crispy and golden brown.
4. Serve the grilled turkey burgers on whole wheat buns with a side of sweet potato fries and a mixed green salad with your favorite dressing.

Spicy Black Bean Soup with Avocado and Salad

Ingredients:

- 2 cans black beans, drained and rinsed
- 1 tablespoon olive oil
- 1 onion, diced
- 2 cloves garlic, minced
- 1 jalapeno pepper, seeded and diced
- 1 red bell pepper, diced
- 1 tablespoon ground cumin
- 1 teaspoon smoked paprika
- 1/4 teaspoon cayenne pepper
- 4 cups low-sodium chicken or vegetable broth
- Salt and pepper to taste
- 1 avocado, diced
- 4 cups mixed greens
- Dressing of choice

Directions:

1. In a large pot, heat the olive oil over medium-high heat. Add the onion, garlic, jalapeno, and red bell pepper, and sauté for 5-7 minutes, until tender.
2. Add the cumin, paprika, and cayenne pepper to the pot and stir to combine. Cook for 1-2 minutes, until fragrant.
3. Add the black beans and chicken or vegetable broth to the pot and bring to a simmer. Simmer for 15-20 minutes, until the soup is hot and the flavors are well combined.
4. Use an immersion blender or transfer the soup to a blender and puree until smooth.

5. Season the soup with salt and pepper to taste.
6. Serve the spicy black bean soup with diced avocado and a mixed green salad with your favorite dressing.

Tips for Success

Here are some tips for success during Week 2 of the Menopause Diet for Weight Loss:

1. Focus on protein-rich foods: Eating foods high in protein, such as lean meats, fish, eggs, and legumes, can help boost your metabolism and keep you feeling full and satisfied throughout the day.
2. Incorporate healthy fats: Healthy fats, such as those found in nuts, seeds, avocados, and olive oil, can help support metabolic function and improve overall health.
3. Stay hydrated: Drinking plenty of water and other hydrating fluids can help support metabolic function and prevent dehydration, which can lead to fatigue and poor digestion.
4. Keep portions in check: Even healthy foods can contribute to weight gain if consumed in excess. Be mindful of portion sizes and aim to fill your plate with a balance of protein, healthy fats, and fiber-rich carbohydrates.
5. Get moving: Regular exercise can help boost your metabolism and support weight loss efforts. Aim for at least 30 minutes of moderate-intensity exercise most days of the week.
6. Prioritize sleep: Adequate sleep is essential for metabolic function and overall health. Aim for 7-9

hours of quality sleep each night to support weight loss and other health goals.

Everyone's body is unique, and it may take time to find the diet and lifestyle habits that work best for you. Be patient, listen to your body, and don't be afraid to make adjustments as needed. With time and dedication, you can achieve your weight loss and menopause symptom management goals.

Chapter 6. Week 3: Reduce Inflammation

During menopause, hormonal changes can lead to increased inflammation in the body, which can contribute to a range of health issues, including weight gain and increased risk of chronic diseases. Week 3 of the Menopause Diet for Weight Loss focuses on reducing inflammation through diet and lifestyle changes.

Daily Meal Plan

Day 15:

Breakfast:

- Avocado toast on whole grain bread with sliced tomato and a sprinkle of red pepper flakes
- Green smoothie with kale, frozen pineapple, almond milk, and protein powder

Snack:

- Hard-boiled egg
- Sliced cucumber with hummus

Lunch:

- Grilled salmon or tofu with roasted Brussels sprouts and quinoa
- Mixed greens salad with cherry tomatoes, cucumber, and a drizzle of olive oil and lemon juice

Snack:

- Apple slices with almond butter
- Handful of almonds

Dinner:

- Lentil and vegetable soup with a slice of whole grain bread
- Steamed green beans with garlic and lemon

Snack:

- Greek yogurt with mixed berries and a sprinkle of cinnamon
- Dark chocolate-covered almonds

Day 16:

Breakfast:

- Greek yogurt with sliced strawberries, granola, and honey
- Green smoothie with spinach, frozen berries, almond milk, and protein powder

Snack:

- Carrot sticks with hummus
- Handful of walnuts

Lunch:

- Grilled chicken or tofu salad with mixed greens, cherry tomatoes, cucumber, and a drizzle of olive oil and balsamic vinegar
- Lentil soup with mixed vegetables and a slice of whole grain bread

Snack:

- Pear slices with almond butter
- Hard-boiled egg

Dinner:

- Turmeric roasted chicken with roasted sweet potato wedges and steamed broccoli
- Quinoa and vegetable stir-fry with ginger and garlic

Snack:

- Greek yogurt with mixed berries and a sprinkle of cinnamon
- Dark chocolate-covered almonds

Day 17:

Breakfast:

- Spinach and feta omelette with whole grain toast
- Green smoothie with kale, frozen mango, almond milk, and protein powder

Snack:

- Sliced cucumber with hummus

- Handful of cashews

Lunch:

- Grilled salmon or tofu with roasted Brussels sprouts and quinoa
- Mixed greens salad with cherry tomatoes, cucumber, and a drizzle of olive oil and lemon juice

Snack:

- Apple slices with almond butter
- Hard-boiled egg

Dinner:

- Baked sweet potato topped with black beans, salsa, and avocado
- Steamed green beans with garlic and lemon

Snack:

- Greek yogurt with mixed berries and a sprinkle of cinnamon
- Dark chocolate-covered almonds

Day 18:

Breakfast:

- Greek yogurt with mixed berries, granola, and honey
- Green smoothie with spinach, frozen peaches, almond milk, and protein powder

Snack:

- Carrot sticks with hummus
- Handful of almonds

Lunch:

- Grilled chicken or tofu salad with mixed greens, cherry tomatoes, cucumber, and a drizzle of olive oil and balsamic vinegar
- Lentil soup with mixed vegetables and a slice of whole grain bread

Snack:

- Pear slices with almond butter
- Hard-boiled egg

Dinner:

- Grilled salmon with roasted asparagus and brown rice
- Quinoa and vegetable stir-fry with ginger and garlic

Snack:

- Greek yogurt with mixed berries and a sprinkle of cinnamon
- Dark chocolate-covered almonds

Day 19:

Breakfast:

- Whole grain toast with avocado and sliced tomato
- Green smoothie with kale, frozen pineapple, almond milk, and protein powder

Snack:

- Handful of walnuts
- Sliced cucumber with hummus

Lunch:

- Grilled chicken or tofu salad with mixed greens, cherry tomatoes, cucumber, and a drizzle of olive oil and lemon juice
- Lentil soup with mixed vegetables and a slice of whole grain bread

Snack:

- Apple slices with almond butter
- Hard-boiled egg

Dinner:

- Baked salmon with roasted Brussels sprouts and sweet potato wedges
- Quinoa and vegetable stir-fry with ginger and garlic

Snack:

- Greek yogurt with mixed berries and a sprinkle of cinnamon
- Dark chocolate-covered almonds

Day 20:

Breakfast:

- Greek yogurt with sliced strawberries, granola, and honey
- Green smoothie with spinach, frozen berries, almond milk, and protein powder

Snack:

- Carrot sticks with hummus
- Handful of almonds

Lunch:

- Grilled chicken or tofu salad with mixed greens, cherry tomatoes, cucumber, and a drizzle of olive oil and balsamic vinegar
- Lentil soup with mixed vegetables and a slice of whole grain bread

Snack:

- Pear slices with almond butter
- Hard-boiled egg

Dinner:

- Turmeric roasted chicken with roasted sweet potato wedges and steamed broccoli
- Quinoa and vegetable stir-fry with ginger and garlic

Snack:

- Greek yogurt with mixed berries and a sprinkle of cinnamon
- Dark chocolate-covered almonds

Day 21:

Breakfast:

- Spinach and feta omelette with whole grain toast
- Green smoothie with kale, frozen mango, almond milk, and protein powder

Snack:

- Sliced cucumber with hummus
- Handful of cashews

Lunch:

- Grilled salmon or tofu with roasted Brussels sprouts and quinoa
- Mixed greens salad with cherry tomatoes, cucumber, and a drizzle of olive oil and lemon juice

Snack:

- Apple slices with almond butter
- Hard-boiled egg

Dinner:

- Baked sweet potato topped with black beans, salsa, and avocado
- Steamed green beans with garlic and lemon

Snack:

- Greek yogurt with mixed berries and a sprinkle of cinnamon
- Dark chocolate-covered almonds

Stay hydrated throughout the day by drinking plenty of water and herbal teas, and aim to get at least 30 minutes of moderate exercise daily to complement your Menopause Diet for Weight Loss.

Recipes and Meal Ideas

Lentil and Vegetable Soup

Ingredients:

- 1 cup lentils
- 1 onion, chopped
- 2 garlic cloves, minced
- 2 carrots, chopped
- 2 celery stalks, chopped
- 1 teaspoon dried thyme
- 1 teaspoon dried oregano
- 1 teaspoon ground cumin
- 6 cups low-sodium vegetable broth
- Salt and pepper to taste
- Lemon wedges for serving

Directions:

1. In a large pot, sauté the onion and garlic over medium heat until fragrant.

2. Add the carrots and celery and continue to sauté for a few more minutes.
3. Add the lentils, thyme, oregano, cumin, and vegetable broth. Bring to a boil.
4. Reduce heat and let the soup simmer for 25-30 minutes, or until the lentils are tender.
5. Season with salt and pepper to taste.
6. Serve with a squeeze of lemon juice.

Turmeric Roasted Chicken

Ingredients:

- 4 chicken breasts
- 1 tablespoon turmeric powder
- 1 teaspoon cumin powder
- 1 teaspoon coriander powder
- 1 teaspoon garlic powder
- Salt and pepper to taste
- 2 tablespoons olive oil
- Lemon wedges for serving

Directions:

1. Preheat the oven to 400°F.
2. In a small bowl, mix together the turmeric, cumin, coriander, garlic powder, salt, and pepper.
3. Rub the spice mixture onto both sides of the chicken breasts.
4. Place the chicken on a baking sheet and drizzle with olive oil.

5. Bake for 25-30 minutes, or until the chicken is cooked through.
6. Serve with lemon wedges.

Quinoa and Vegetable Stir-Fry

Ingredients:

- 1 cup quinoa
- 2 cups low-sodium vegetable broth
- 1 tablespoon olive oil
- 1 onion, chopped
- 2 garlic cloves, minced
- 1 red bell pepper, chopped
- 1 yellow bell pepper, chopped
- 2 cups broccoli florets
- 1 tablespoon ginger, grated
- 2 tablespoons low-sodium soy sauce
- Salt and pepper to taste

Directions:

1. Rinse the quinoa and place it in a pot with the vegetable broth. Bring to a boil.
2. Reduce heat and let the quinoa simmer for 15-20 minutes, or until the liquid is absorbed.
3. In a large pan, heat the olive oil over medium heat.
4. Add the onion and garlic and sauté for a few minutes.

5. Add the bell peppers, broccoli, and ginger and continue to sauté for 5-7 minutes, or until the vegetables are tender.
6. Add the cooked quinoa and soy sauce to the pan and stir to combine.
7. Season with salt and pepper to taste.

Grilled Salmon with Quinoa and Roasted Brussels Sprouts

Ingredients:

- 4 salmon fillets
- Salt and pepper to taste
- 2 tablespoons lemon juice
- 1 cup quinoa
- 2 cups low-sodium vegetable broth
- 1 pound Brussels sprouts, trimmed and halved
- 2 tablespoons olive oil
- Salt and pepper to taste

Directions:

1. Preheat the grill to medium-high heat.
2. Season the salmon fillets with salt, pepper, and lemon juice.
3. Grill the salmon for 3-4 minutes per side, or until cooked through.
4. Rinse the quinoa and place it in a pot with the vegetable broth. Bring to a boil.
5. Reduce heat and let the quinoa simmer for 15-20 minutes, or until the liquid is absorbed.

6. Meanwhile, toss the Brussels sprouts with olive oil, salt, and pepper, and spread them in a single layer on a baking sheet. Roast in the oven at 400°F for 20-25 minutes, or until tender and lightly browned.
7. Serve the grilled salmon with the cooked quinoa and roasted Brussels sprouts.

Lentil and Vegetable Stir-Fry

Ingredients:

- 1 cup lentils
- 2 cups low-sodium vegetable broth
- 1 tablespoon olive oil
- 1 onion, chopped
- 2 garlic cloves, minced
- 1 red bell pepper, chopped
- 1 yellow bell pepper, chopped
- 2 cups broccoli florets
- 1 tablespoon ginger, grated
- 2 tablespoons low-sodium soy sauce
- Salt and pepper to taste

Directions:

1. Rinse the lentils and place them in a pot with the vegetable broth. Bring to a boil.
2. Reduce heat and let the lentils simmer for 25-30 minutes, or until tender.
3. In a large pan, heat the olive oil over medium heat.
4. Add the onion and garlic and sauté for a few minutes.

5. Add the bell peppers, broccoli, and ginger and continue to sauté for 5-7 minutes, or until the vegetables are tender.
6. Add the cooked lentils and soy sauce to the pan and stir to combine.
7. Season with salt and pepper to taste.

Tips for Success

Here are some tips for success during Week 3:

1. Choose anti-inflammatory foods: Incorporate foods that are rich in anti-inflammatory nutrients like omega-3 fatty acids, vitamin C, and turmeric into your meals. Examples include salmon, walnuts, leafy greens, berries, and ginger.
2. Limit processed foods: Processed foods can be high in added sugars and unhealthy fats, which can contribute to inflammation. Focus on whole foods instead.
3. Incorporate herbs and spices: Adding herbs and spices to your meals can not only add flavor, but also provide anti-inflammatory benefits. Try adding fresh herbs like basil, parsley, and cilantro, and spices like turmeric and cumin.
4. Stay hydrated: Drinking plenty of water can help flush toxins from your body and reduce inflammation. Aim for at least 8 cups of water per day.
5. Be mindful of food sensitivities: Some people may have food sensitivities that can contribute to inflammation. Pay attention to how your body

reacts to certain foods and avoid those that cause negative symptoms.

Incorporating these tips and anti-inflammatory foods into your diet can help reduce inflammation in your body, promoting better health and well-being.

Chapter 7. Week 4: Maintain and Sustain

Maintain and Sustain is an important part of the Menopause Diet for Weight Loss program. This week is designed to help you build on the progress you've made during the first three weeks of the program and establish healthy habits that will last long after the program has ended.

The daily meal plan is designed to provide a balanced and sustainable approach to eating. This plan emphasizes whole foods, lean proteins, and healthy fats, while minimizing processed foods and added sugars. By following this plan, you can continue to fuel your body with nutrient-dense foods that support weight loss and overall health.

Week 4 includes a variety of delicious and healthy recipes designed to be easy to prepare and incorporate into a busy lifestyle, making it easy to continue eating healthily long after the program has ended.

Daily Meal Plan

Day 22

Breakfast:

- Smoothie bowl with mixed berries, banana, spinach, and almond butter
- Whole grain toast with avocado and sliced tomato

Snack:

- Greek yogurt with sliced peaches and honey
- Small handful of almonds

Lunch:

- Roasted vegetable quinoa bowl with hummus and lemon-tahini dressing
- Side salad with mixed greens, cherry tomatoes, and balsamic vinaigrette

Snack:

- Cut veggies with hummus
- Small piece of dark chocolate

Dinner:

- Baked chicken with roasted sweet potatoes and green beans
- Side salad with mixed greens, cucumber, and vinaigrette

Snack:

- Sliced apple with almond butter
- Hard boiled egg

Day 23

Breakfast:

- Omelet with spinach, mushrooms, and feta cheese
- Whole grain toast with jam

Snack:

- Greek yogurt with mixed berries and granola
- Small handful of cashews

Lunch:

- Tuna salad with mixed greens, cherry tomatoes, and vinaigrette
- Side of roasted Brussels sprouts

Snack:

- Raw veggies with hummus
- Small piece of dark chocolate

Dinner:

- Grilled shrimp skewers with roasted vegetables and quinoa
- Side salad with mixed greens and vinaigrette

Snack:

- Sliced pear with cheese
- Handful of grapes

Day 24

Breakfast:

- Greek yogurt with sliced strawberries and honey
- Whole grain toast with almond butter

Snack:

- Celery sticks with hummus
- Small handful of walnuts

Lunch:

- Smoked salmon with whole grain crackers, sliced cucumber, and cream cheese
- Side salad with mixed greens and vinaigrette

Snack:

- Cut veggies with hummus
- Small piece of dark chocolate

Dinner:

- Baked salmon with roasted asparagus and brown rice
- Side salad with mixed greens and vinaigrette

Snack:

- Sliced apple with almond butter
- Small handful of almonds

Day 25

Breakfast:

- Smoothie with mixed berries, banana, spinach, and protein powder
- Whole grain toast with avocado and sliced tomato

Snack:

- Greek yogurt with mixed berries and granola
- Small handful of cashews

Lunch:

- Grilled chicken with mixed greens, cherry tomatoes, and vinaigrette
- Side of roasted sweet potato wedges

Snack:

- Cut veggies with hummus
- Small piece of dark chocolate

Dinner:

- Turkey meatballs with whole grain pasta and roasted vegetables
- Side salad with mixed greens and vinaigrette

Snack:

- Sliced pear with cheese
- Handful of grapes

Day 26

Breakfast:

- Omelet with spinach, mushrooms, and goat cheese
- Whole grain toast with jam

Snack:

- Greek yogurt with sliced peaches and honey
- Small handful of almonds

Lunch:

- Grilled chicken Caesar salad with whole grain croutons
- Side of roasted vegetables

Snack:

- Cut veggies with hummus
- Small piece of dark chocolate

Dinner:

- Grilled salmon with roasted Brussels sprouts and quinoa
- Side salad with mixed greens and vinaigrette

Snack:

- Sliced apple with almond butter
- Hard boiled egg

Day 27

Breakfast:

- Smoothie bowl with mixed berries, banana, spinach, and almond butter
- Whole grain toast with avocado and sliced tomato

Snack:

- Greek yogurt with mixed berries and granola
- Small handful of cashews

Lunch:

- Turkey and avocado wrap with mixed greens and hummus
- Side of cut veggies

Snack:

- Raw veggies with hummus
- Small piece of dark chocolate

Dinner:

- Grilled chicken with roasted sweet potatoes and green beans
- Side salad with mixed greens and vinaigrette

Snack:

- Sliced pear with cheese
- Handful of grapes

Day 28

Breakfast:

- Greek yogurt with sliced strawberries and honey
- Whole grain toast with almond butter

Snack:

- Celery sticks with hummus
- Small handful of walnuts

Lunch:

- Grilled shrimp with mixed greens, cherry tomatoes, and vinaigrette
- Side of roasted vegetables

Snack:

- Cut veggies with hummus
- Small piece of dark chocolate

Dinner:

- Baked chicken with roasted asparagus and quinoa
- Side salad with mixed greens and vinaigrette

Snack:

- Sliced apple with almond butter
- Small handful of almonds

Listen to your body's hunger and fullness signals throughout the day. Enjoy!

Day 29 and 30 (Flex days)

Prioritizing self-care is an essential part of any successful weight loss plan. The two remaining days in the 30-Day Menopause Diet Plan for Weight Loss offer the perfect opportunity to prioritize self-care and take a break from the demands of daily life.

Self-care can take many forms, including meditation, journaling, spending time in nature, getting a massage, or simply taking a relaxing bath. These activities help to reduce stress, promote relaxation, and boost mood, all of which are crucial for supporting overall health and well-being.

On flex days, make sure to take some time for yourself and engage in activities that make you feel good. This could be as simple as taking a walk in nature or listening to your favorite music. Whatever you choose to do, make sure it supports your overall health and well-being.

Prioritizing self-care on flex days also helps to reduce the risk of burnout and exhaustion, which can impede your weight loss goals. By taking care of yourself, you'll have more energy and motivation to stick to your healthy habits and continue making progress toward your goals.

Make the most of your two remaining days by prioritizing self-care and engaging in activities that support your overall health and well-being. Remember, taking care of yourself is an essential part of any successful weight loss journey.

Recipes and Meal Ideas

Roasted Vegetable Quinoa Bowl with Hummus and Lemon-Tahini Dressing

Ingredients:

- 1 cup quinoa
- 2 cups low-sodium vegetable broth
- 1 red bell pepper, sliced
- 1 zucchini, sliced
- 1 yellow squash, sliced
- 1 tablespoon olive oil
- Salt and pepper to taste
- 1/4 cup hummus
- 2 tablespoons lemon juice
- 2 tablespoons tahini
- 1 clove garlic, minced
- 1/4 teaspoon ground cumin
- Water as needed

Directions:

1. Preheat the oven to 425°F.
2. In a medium saucepan, bring quinoa and vegetable broth to a boil. Reduce heat to low, cover, and simmer for 15-20 minutes, or until quinoa is cooked through.
3. Toss sliced bell pepper, zucchini, and yellow squash with olive oil, salt, and pepper, and spread in a single

layer on a baking sheet. Roast for 15-20 minutes, until vegetables are tender and lightly browned.

4. In a small bowl, whisk together hummus, lemon juice, tahini, garlic, cumin, and enough water to thin to a dressing consistency.

5. To assemble, divide cooked quinoa and roasted vegetables among four bowls. Drizzle with lemon-tahini dressing and serve.

Baked Chicken with Roasted Sweet Potatoes and Green Beans

Ingredients:

- 4 boneless, skinless chicken breasts
- 1 tablespoon olive oil
- Salt and pepper to taste
- 2 large sweet potatoes, peeled and diced
- 1 pound fresh green beans, trimmed
- 2 tablespoons balsamic vinegar
- 2 tablespoons honey
- 2 tablespoons Dijon mustard

Directions:

1. Preheat the oven to 400°F.
2. Place chicken breasts in a baking dish and drizzle with olive oil. Season with salt and pepper.
3. Toss diced sweet potatoes and green beans with olive oil, salt, and pepper, and spread in a single layer on a baking sheet.

4. Bake chicken and vegetables for 20-25 minutes, or until chicken is cooked through and vegetables are tender.
5. In a small bowl, whisk together balsamic vinegar, honey, and Dijon mustard.
6. To serve, divide chicken, sweet potatoes, and green beans among four plates. Drizzle with balsamic honey mustard sauce.

Tuna Salad with Mixed Greens, Cherry Tomatoes, and Vinaigrette

Ingredients:

- 2 cans tuna, drained
- 1/4 cup chopped red onion
- 1/4 cup chopped celery
- 1/4 cup plain Greek yogurt
- 2 tablespoons lemon juice
- 1 tablespoon Dijon mustard
- Salt and pepper to taste
- 4 cups mixed greens
- 1 cup cherry tomatoes, halved
- 2 tablespoons red wine vinegar
- 2 tablespoons olive oil

Directions:

1. In a large bowl, combine tuna, red onion, celery, Greek yogurt, lemon juice, Dijon mustard, salt, and pepper. Mix well and set aside.

2. In a separate bowl, combine mixed greens and cherry tomatoes.
3. In a small bowl, whisk together red wine vinegar, olive oil, salt, and pepper.
4. To serve, divide tuna salad and mixed greens among four plates. Drizzle with vinaigrette.

Whole Grain Toast with Avocado and Sliced Tomato:

Ingredients:

- 4 slices whole grain bread
- 1 avocado, mashed
- Salt and pepper to taste 4 slices tomato

Directions:

1. Toast the whole grain bread slices.
2. Spread the mashed avocado evenly on each slice of toast.
3. Season with salt and pepper to taste.
4. Top each slice with a slice of tomato.
5. Serve and enjoy.

Tips for Success

To ensure success in maintaining and sustaining the healthy habits you've developed over the past three weeks, here are some tips to keep in mind:

1. Plan ahead: Take time each week to plan out your meals and snacks for the upcoming week. This will

help you stay on track and avoid making unhealthy food choices out of convenience.

2. Keep healthy snacks on hand: Stock your pantry and fridge with healthy snacks like fruits, vegetables, nuts, and seeds. This will help you avoid reaching for unhealthy snacks when you're feeling hungry.

3. Practice mindful eating: Remember to slow down and savor your meals, paying attention to how your body feels as you eat. This can help prevent overeating and promote better digestion.

4. Stay hydrated: Make sure to drink plenty of water throughout the day to stay hydrated and help flush toxins out of your body.

5. Be kind to yourself: Remember that sustainable change takes time and effort, and that it's okay to slip up occasionally. Don't beat yourself up over a small setback, but rather use it as motivation to continue making positive changes.

Chapter 8. Exercise and Lifestyle Changes

In addition to following the 30-Day Menopause Diet Plan for Weight Loss, incorporating regular exercise and lifestyle changes is crucial for achieving long-term weight loss and overall health.

Types of Exercise for Menopausal Women

There are several types of exercise that are particularly beneficial for menopausal women, including:

1. Strength training: Strength training helps to build lean muscle mass, which can increase metabolism and support weight loss. It also supports bone health, reducing the risk of osteoporosis.
2. Cardiovascular exercise: Cardiovascular exercise, such as walking, jogging, or cycling, helps to burn calories and improve cardiovascular health.
3. Yoga or Pilates: These types of exercise support flexibility, balance, and core strength, and can also reduce stress and promote relaxation.

The Benefits of Exercise during Menopause

Exercise is crucial for menopausal women to maintain good health and reduce the risk of chronic diseases. Here are some of the key benefits of regular exercise during menopause:

1. Weight Management: As metabolism slows down during menopause, regular exercise can help to maintain a healthy weight and reduce the risk of obesity.
2. Cardiovascular Health: Regular exercise can improve heart health by lowering blood pressure, reducing the risk of heart disease, and decreasing LDL cholesterol levels.
3. Bone Health: Menopausal women are at an increased risk of osteoporosis, but weight-bearing exercises such as walking, running, or weightlifting can help to maintain bone density.
4. Mood and Mental Health: Exercise has been shown to reduce symptoms of depression and anxiety and improve overall mood during menopause.
5. Sleep Quality: Regular exercise can improve sleep quality and duration, which is especially important for menopausal women who may experience disrupted sleep.
6. Hormone Regulation: Exercise can help regulate hormone levels during menopause, reducing symptoms such as hot flashes and night sweats.

Incorporating regular exercise into your menopause diet for weight loss plan is essential for maintaining good health and reducing the risk of chronic diseases. Even small amounts of physical activity can have significant health benefits, so find an activity that you enjoy and try to incorporate it into your daily routine.

Simple Exercise Routines to Incorporate into Your Day (exercise plan)

here's a simple exercise routine for each day of the week to help you incorporate physical activity into your day:

Day 1: Cardiovascular Exercise

- Brisk walk or jog for 30 minutes
- Jumping jacks for 3 sets of 10 reps
- Burpees for 3 sets of 10 reps

Day 2: Strength Training

- Squats for 3 sets of 10 reps
- Push-ups for 3 sets of 10 reps
- Lunges for 3 sets of 10 reps
- Plank for 30 seconds, rest for 30 seconds, repeat for 3 sets

Day 3: Yoga and Stretching

- Sun salutations for 3 sets of 10 reps
- Warrior 2 pose for 3 sets of 30 seconds on each side
- Downward dog for 3 sets of 30 seconds
- Child's pose for 3 sets of 30 seconds

Day 4: Pilates

- The hundred for 3 sets of 10 reps

- The roll-up for 3 sets of 10 reps
- The single-leg stretch for 3 sets of 10 reps on each leg
- The plank for 30 seconds, rest for 30 seconds, repeat for 3 sets

Day 5: Interval Training

- Warm up with 5 minutes of light cardio (e.g., jumping jacks)
- Sprint for 30 seconds, rest for 30 seconds, repeat for 10 sets
- Jump rope for 3 sets of 1 minute
- Cool down with 5 minutes of light cardio (e.g., walking)

Day 6: Total Body Workout

- Burpees for 3 sets of 10 reps
- Push-ups for 3 sets of 10 reps
- Squats for 3 sets of 10 reps
- Lunges for 3 sets of 10 reps on each leg
- Plank for 30 seconds, rest for 30 seconds, and repeat for 3 sets

Day 7: Rest and Recovery

- Take the day off to rest and recover from your workouts
- Do gentle activities like walking, yoga, or stretching
- Focus on getting enough sleep, staying hydrated, and nourishing your body with healthy foods

Listen to your body and adjust the intensity and duration of your workouts as needed. Consistency is key when it comes to exercise, so aim to incorporate physical activity into your daily routine and make it a habit. With regular exercise and a healthy menopause diet for weight loss, you can improve your overall health and well-being and manage menopause symptoms more effectively.

Lifestyle Changes for Optimal Health and Weight Loss
Making lifestyle changes is an essential part of any successful weight loss and health program. As you navigate through menopause, it's important to incorporate habits that can help you achieve optimal health and maintain a healthy weight. Here are some lifestyle changes you can implement:

1. Stay hydrated: Drinking enough water is essential for overall health and can help reduce bloating, constipation, and fatigue. Aim to drink at least 8 cups of water per day, and more if you exercise or live in a hot climate.
2. Get enough sleep: Lack of sleep can disrupt hormone balance, increase stress levels, and make weight loss more challenging. Aim for 7-8 hours of

sleep per night to support your overall health and well-being.

3. Manage stress: High stress levels can trigger menopause symptoms and make weight loss more challenging. Try relaxation techniques like yoga, meditation, or deep breathing to reduce stress and promote relaxation.

4. Practice self-care: Taking time for yourself and engaging in activities you enjoy can help reduce stress and support emotional well-being. Consider hobbies like reading, painting, or taking a relaxing bath to prioritize self-care.

5. Limit alcohol and processed foods: These items can be high in calories and negatively impact overall health. Limiting or eliminating these from your diet can support weight loss and overall health.

Incorporating these lifestyle changes alongside a healthy menopause diet for weight loss and regular exercise can help you achieve optimal health and manage menopause symptoms more effectively.

Chapter 9. Conclusion

Congratulations on completing the 30-day menopause diet for weight loss! This is a significant achievement, and you should be proud of yourself for the hard work and dedication you have put in.

Take a moment to reflect on how far you have come in just 30 days. You have learned about the benefits of a menopause diet, experimented with new recipes, and incorporated exercise and self-care into your daily routine.

Now is the time to celebrate your successes. Whether you lost weight, improved your energy levels, or reduced your menopause symptoms, these are all significant achievements that deserve recognition.

Consider treating yourself to something special as a reward for your hard work. It could be a spa day, a new outfit, or a weekend getaway. Whatever it is, make sure it's something that brings you joy and helps you feel proud of yourself.

Remember that this journey is not just about the 30 days, but about making long-term lifestyle changes that will support your health and well-being. Use the momentum from your successes to keep pushing forward and making progress towards your goals.

And finally, don't forget to give yourself credit for the effort you have put in. Even on days when things felt challenging or overwhelming, you showed up and did your best. Celebrate your successes, no matter how small, and use them as motivation to keep moving forward towards a healthier, happier you.

Continuing Your Menopause Diet for Long-Term Health and Wellness.

As you approach the end of your 30-day menopause diet plan, it's important to remember that the changes you've made to your eating habits and lifestyle are not just temporary measures, but rather a foundation for long-term health and wellness. In this section, we'll discuss strategies for continuing your menopause diet and incorporating healthy habits into your everyday life.

1. Make a plan: Take some time to think about your long-term health goals and how you can continue to make progress towards them. Create a plan for your diet and exercise routine, setting achievable goals for yourself and outlining the steps you need to take to reach them.

2. Keep it interesting: One of the keys to sticking with any healthy habit is to keep things interesting and enjoyable. Continue to experiment with new recipes and ingredients, try different forms of exercise, and find ways to incorporate movement into your daily routine.

3. Find a support system: Having a supportive network of family, friends, or even online communities can be invaluable in helping you stay on track and motivated. Reach out to others who share your goals and challenges, and lean on them for support and encouragement.

4. Monitor your progress: Keep track of your progress towards your long-term health goals, and celebrate your successes along the way. Whether it's losing a few pounds, running a 5k, or simply feeling more energized and healthy, take the time to acknowledge your achievements and use them as motivation to keep going.

5. Practice self-compassion: Remember that maintaining a healthy lifestyle is not always easy, and that setbacks and challenges are a natural part of the process. Be kind to yourself, practice self-compassion, and focus on the positive changes you've made and the progress you've already achieved.

By incorporating these strategies into your daily life, you can continue to reap the benefits of your menopause diet and achieve long-term health and wellness.

Resources

Shopping List

Creating a shopping list is an essential part of any successful menopause diet plan for weight loss. Here are some items to add to your grocery list to support your weight loss and overall health goals during menopause:

1. Fresh fruits and vegetables: Aim for a variety of colorful produce to get a range of vitamins, minerals, and antioxidants. Some great options include leafy greens, berries, citrus fruits, cruciferous vegetables, and sweet potatoes.
2. Lean proteins: Choose lean protein sources like chicken, turkey, fish, tofu, and legumes to support muscle health and promote fullness.
3. Whole grains: Opt for whole grains like quinoa, brown rice, and whole wheat bread instead of refined grains to provide more fiber and nutrients.
4. Nuts and seeds: These can provide healthy fats, protein, and fiber. Try incorporating almonds, chia seeds, flaxseeds, or pumpkin seeds into your meals or snacks.
5. Healthy fats: Incorporate sources of healthy fats like avocado, olive oil, nuts, and seeds to support brain health and reduce inflammation.
6. Low-fat dairy or dairy alternatives: These can provide important nutrients like calcium and vitamin D. Consider options like skim milk, Greek yogurt, or almond milk.

Remember to adjust your shopping list based on your individual dietary needs and preferences. Using a shopping list can help you stay organized and focused when grocery shopping, and ensure that you have healthy options on hand to support your weight loss and overall health goals during menopause.

Glossary of Terms

Here are 20 key terms related to menopause and weight loss that you may come across when following the 30-day menopause diet plan:

1. Menopause: The time in a woman's life when her menstrual periods stop, typically occurring between the ages of 45-55.
2. Perimenopause: The period leading up to menopause, during which a woman may experience irregular periods and other symptoms.
3. Hormone replacement therapy (HRT): Medications used to supplement the body's declining levels of estrogen and progesterone during menopause.
4. Hot flashes: Sudden sensations of heat that may cause sweating, flushing, and rapid heartbeat.
5. Night sweats: Episodes of sweating during sleep, often associated with menopause.
6. Visceral fat: Fat that accumulates around the internal organs and can contribute to health problems like heart disease and diabetes.
7. Basal metabolic rate (BMR): The number of calories the body burns at rest.
8. Lean body mass: The weight of the body's bones, muscles, and organs, not including fat.
9. Resistance training: Exercises that use weights, resistance bands, or body weight to build strength and muscle mass.

10. Cardiovascular exercise: Activities like running, swimming, or cycling that increase heart rate and improve cardiovascular health.
11. High-intensity interval training (HIIT): Short bursts of intense exercise followed by periods of rest or low-intensity exercise.
12. Insulin resistance: A condition in which the body's cells become resistant to the hormone insulin, which can lead to high blood sugar levels and other health problems.
13. Glycemic index (GI): A measure of how quickly a food raises blood sugar levels.
14. Fiber: A type of carbohydrate that the body cannot digest, found in fruits, vegetables, and whole grains.
15. Phytoestrogens: Plant compounds that can mimic the effects of estrogen in the body.
16. Cortisol: A hormone produced by the body in response to stress, which can contribute to weight gain and other health problems.
17. Mindfulness: A state of focused awareness and non-judgmental acceptance of the present moment.
18. Sleep hygiene: The practices and habits that promote good quality sleep.
19. Self-care: Actions taken to improve one's physical, mental, and emotional well-being.
20. Motivation: The drive or desire to achieve a goal, often influenced by internal and external factors.

Additional Reading and References

1. The Menopause Book: The Complete Guide to Managing Your Symptoms and Improving Your Well-Being by Barbara Kantrowitz and Pat Wingert
2. The Menopause Answer Book: Practical Answers, Treatments, and Solutions for Your Unique Symptoms by Dr. Marsha Nunley
3. The Wisdom of Menopause Journal by Dr. Christiane Northrup
4. The Secret Pleasures of Menopause by Dr. Christiane Northrup
5. Menopause Without Medicine: The Trusted Women's Resource with the Latest Information on HRT, Breast Cancer, Heart Disease, and Natural Alternatives by Linda Ojeda

Printed in Great Britain
by Amazon

32294644R00055